Mastering Dental Assisting

Essential Skills and Techniques for Dental Professionals"

Lula Nicolas

Table of Contents:
Introduction

Overview of Dental Assistance

Dental assistants' role:

Introduction

Overview of Dental Assistance

In the realm of dentistry, dental assisting is a vibrant and essential career that involves a variety of vital duties that support a dental practice's overall productivity and success. As essential part of the oral healthcare team, dental assistants help dentists by supporting them and making sure patients receive high-quality care. The purpose of this introduction is to describe the diverse responsibilities of dental assistants and highlight their importance within the field of dental treatment.

1. Dental assistants' role:

Dental assistants are vital members of the team that support dentists in a variety of clinical and administrative capacities. Sterilizing equipment, setting up treatment areas, and making sure everything runs smoothly are all part of their duties Chairside dental assistants are essential.

Chapter one

Patient Communication:

Effective Communication Skills:
Developing strong interpersonal skills to establish rapport and trust with patients.
Active listening techniques to understand patient concerns and address them effectively.
Educational Communication:

Communicating dental procedures and treatment plans in a clear and understandable manner.
Providing patients with oral hygiene instructions and preventive care information.

Empathy and Compassion:
Understanding the emotional aspects of dental care and demonstrating empathy towards anxious or nervous patients.

Communicating with sensitivity, particularly when discussing treatment options and outcomes.

Crisis Communication:

Handling patient emergencies with composure and clarity.
Effectively communicating unexpected complications or changes in treatment plans.

Infection Control:

Cross-contamination Prevention:
Rigorous adherence to sterilization protocols for instruments and equipment.
Proper disposal of contaminated materials and adherence to universal precautions.

Personal Protective Equipment (PPE):
Proper selection and use of PPE, including gloves, masks, and eyewear.

Training on donning and doffing PPE to minimize the risk of infection transmission.

Environmental Infection Control:
Regular disinfection of surfaces and equipment in treatment areas.
Maintenance of a clean and hygienic dental office environment.

Patient and Staff Education:
Educating patients on infection control measures and the importance of a sterile environment.
Training dental staff on infection prevention best practices and updates.Dental Anatomy and Tooth Identification:

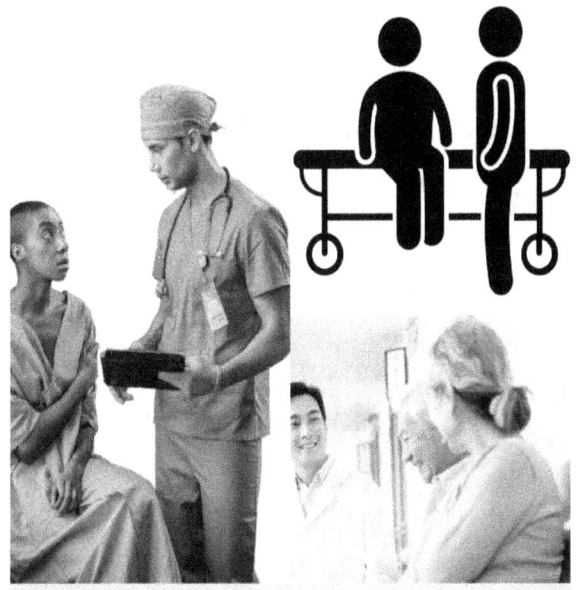
Comtion scenarious with patients

Chapter two

Dental Anatomy and tooth identification:

Tooth Morphology:

Understanding the anatomy of different tooth types, including incisors, canines, premolars, and molars.
Recognition of tooth surfaces and their functions in the chewing process.

Oral Structures:

Knowledge of oral cavity structures, such as the gingiva, palate, and tongue.
Understanding the relationship between oral structures and their impact on dental health.

Tooth Numbering and Charting:

Proficiency in tooth numbering systems (e.g., Universal, Palmer) for accurate charting.
Ability to identify and document dental conditions and treatments through charting.

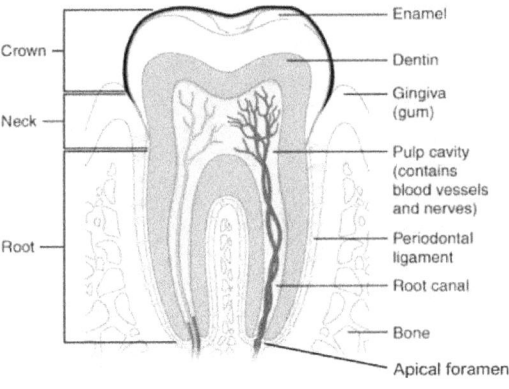

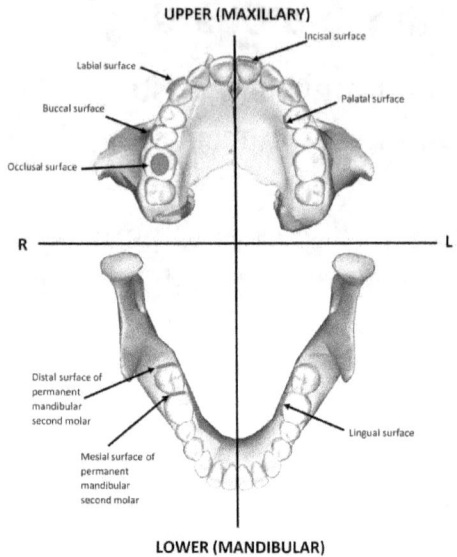

UPPER (MAXILLARY)

Incisal surface

Labial surface

Buccal surface

Palatal surface

Occlusal surface

R ———————————————— L

Distal surface of
permanent
mandibular
second molar

Lingual surface

Mesial surface of
permanent
mandibular
second molar

LOWER (MANDIBULAR)

13

Clinical Application:

Applying knowledge of dental anatomy during chairside assistance in various dental procedures.
Recognizing abnormalities or variations in tooth anatomy that may impact treatment planning.
These topics are integral components of dental assisting, and a thorough understanding of each contributes to the overall competency and professionalism of dental healthcare practitioners.
Tooth Surfaces and Types:

Incisors:
Location: Found at the front of the mouth.
Function: Cutting and biting; essential for initial food breakdown.

Canines:
Location: Pointed teeth adjacent to the incisors.

Function: Grasping and tearing; crucial for tearing food.
Premolars:
Location: Behind the canines.
Function: Crushing and grinding; play a role in breaking down food particles.

Molars:
Location: Located at the back of the mouth.
Function: Grinding and chewing; primary contributors to effective mastication.

Tooth Surfaces:
The chewing surface of the back teeth is called the occlusal.

Buccal Surface: The outer surface facing the cheek.
Lingual Surface: The inner surface facing the tongue.
Mesial Surface: The side of the tooth facing toward the midline.
Distal Surface: The side of the tooth facing away from the midline.

Understanding tooth surfaces and types is essential for dental assistants in facilitating effective communication with dentists, assisting during procedures, and contributing to accurate charting of dental conditions.

Oral Cavity Structures:

Gingiva (Gums):
Function: Surrounds and supports the teeth, providing a protective barrier.
Importance: Healthy gums are crucial for overall oral health and stability of teeth.
Palate:

Hard Palate: Forms the front portion of the roof of the mouth.
Soft Palate: Comprises the back portion and aids in speech and swallowing.

Tongue:

Function: A muscular organ essential for speech, taste, and manipulation of food.
Papillae: Contain taste buds, contributing to the sense of taste.
Salivary Glands:
Function: Produce saliva, aiding in digestion, lubrication, and protection against bacteria.
Major Glands: Parotid, submandibular, and sublingual glands.
Understanding oral cavity structures is foundational for dental assistants in providing effective chairside assistance, educating patients on oral hygiene practices, and contributing to the overall maintenance of oral health.

Chapter three

Dental Instruments and Equipment:

Basic Dental Instruments:
Mirror and Explorer: Essential for visual examination and detection of dental issues.
Scaler and Curette: Used for removing plaque and tartar from teeth.

Chairside Assistance Tools:
Instrument Handling:
 X-ray images.

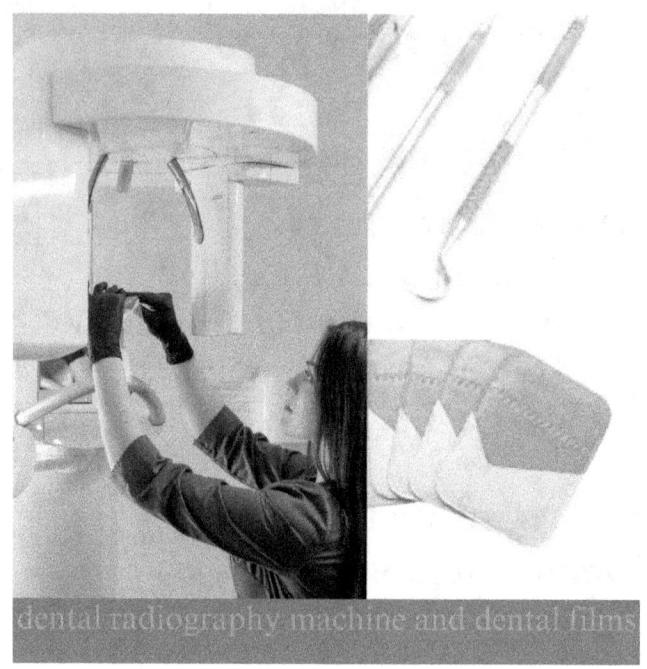

dental radiography machine and dental films

Sterilization Equipment:
Autoclave: Ensures proper sterilization of instruments.
Ultrasonic Cleaner: Removes debris from instruments before sterilization.
Dental assistants must be proficient in the use and maintenance of dental instruments and equipment to ensure a sterile environment, support dentists during procedures, and contribute to the delivery of high-quality patient care.

Common Dental Instruments:

Mirror and Explorer:
Purpose: Visual examination and detection of dental issues.
Use: Reflects light into the oral cavity for better visibility, while the explorer helps identify cavities or irregularities in tooth Surface.

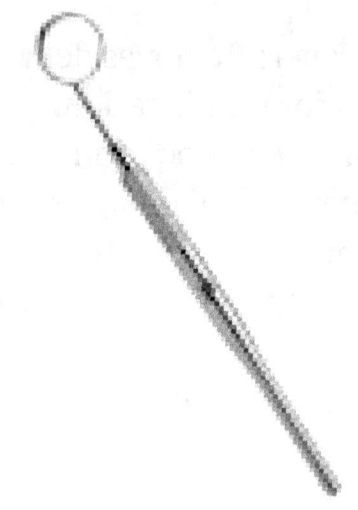

MOUTH MIRRROR

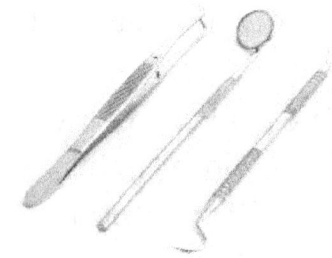

BASIC DENTAL INSTRUMENTS

Scaler and Curette:
Purpose: Removal of plaque and tartar from teeth.
Use: Scalers break down larger deposits, while curettes are designed for finer cleaning along the gumline and root surfaces.

Dental Forceps:
Purpose: Extraction of teeth.
Use: Various forceps are designed for specific teeth and extraction scenarios, ensuring precision and minimal trauma.

Excavators:
Purpose: Removal of decayed tooth structure.
Use: Different excavators are employed for the precise removal of carious material before restorative procedures.

Dental Handpieces:
Purpose: Cutting, polishing, and shaping dental materials.
Types: High-speed handpieces for cutting and low-speed handpieces for polishing and finishing.
Chairside Assistance Tools:
High-Speed and Low-Speed Handpieces:
Use: High-speed for efficient tooth preparation, low-speed for polishing and finishing.
Importance: Facilitate various dental procedures with precision and speed.

Suction Devices:
Purpose: Removal of saliva and debris from the oral cavity.
Use: Ensures a clear operating field for the dentist, enhancing visibility during procedures.

Dental Dam:
Purpose: Isolation of teeth during certain procedures.
Use: Creates a dry field, improving the precision of dental work and preventing contamination.
Matrix Bands and Retainers:
Purpose: Provides a temporary wall for restorative materials.
Use: Creates a form for the placement of fillings, ensuring proper contour and contact.

Dental Radiography:

X-ray Machines:
Purpose: Capturing images of teeth and oral structures for diagnostic purposes.
Types: Intraoral (inside the mouth) and extraoral (outside the mouth) machines.

Digital Sensors or Film:
Purpose: Recording X-ray images.

Advantages: Digital sensors provide instant images with lower radiation exposure compared to traditional film.

Bitewing and Periapical X-rays:
Purpose: Detailed views of specific areas of the mouth.
Use: Detecting cavities, assessing root health, and evaluating bone levels.

Panoramic X-rays:
Purpose: Capturing an overview of the entire oral cavity.
Use: Assessing overall dental health, including impacted teeth, jaw joints, and sinus cavities.
Understanding these common dental instruments, chairside assistance tools, and dental radiography equipment is crucial for dental assistants in providing efficient support during procedures, maintaining a sterile environment, and contributing to accurate diagnostic imaging for patient care.

Amalgamator:
Purpose: Mixing dental amalgam for restorative procedures.
Use: Ensures a homogenous and well-blended amalgam for dental fillings.
Dental Radiography (Continued):

Cone Beam Computed Tomography (CBCT):
Purpose: 3D imaging for detailed views of oral and maxillofacial structures.
Use: Essential for treatment planning in complex cases, such as implant placement and orthodontic assessments.

Radiographic Positioning Tools:
Purpose: Ensuring accurate and consistent positioning of the X-ray equipment and the patient.
Use: Proper positioning minimizes retakes and ensures diagnostic quality images.

Lead Aprons and Thyroid Collars:
Purpose: Radiation protection for patients.
Importance: Shields sensitive body areas
from unnecessary radiation exposure during
X-ray procedures.

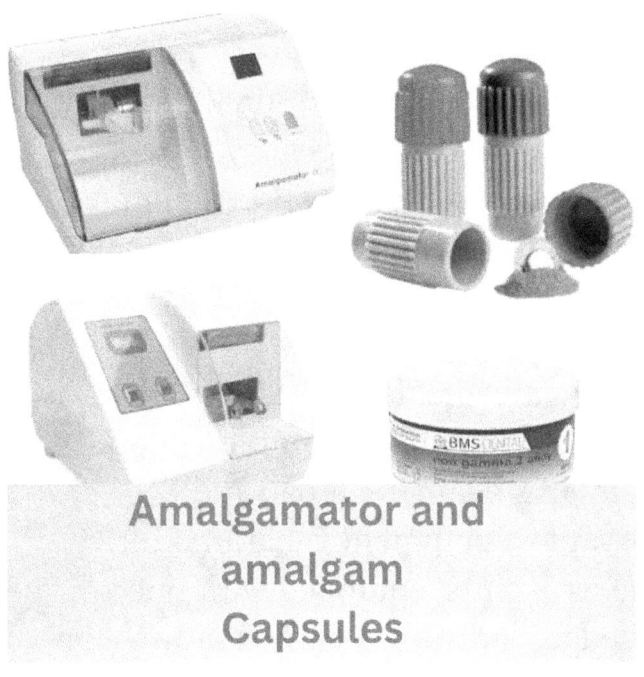

Amalgamator and
amalgam
Capsules

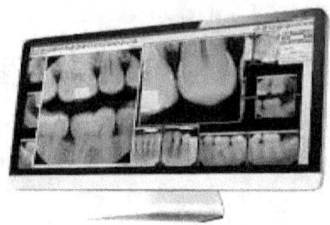

Automatic Film Processors or Digital Imaging Software:

Purpose: Developing traditional X-ray film or managing digital images.

Advantages: Automation speeds up the development process, while digital imaging allows for manipulation and storage of electronic records.

In the dynamic field of dental assisting, proficiency in handling common dental instruments, chairside tools, and radiography equipment is paramount. Dental assistants, equipped with this knowledge, contribute significantly to the delivery of precise and efficient dental care, ensuring patient comfort and optimal oral health outcomes.

Chapter four

X-ray Techniques:

Intraoral X-rays:
Purpose: Capturing detailed images of individual teeth and surrounding structures.
Techniques: Bitewing for interproximal areas, periapical for entire tooth structure, occlusal for large areas of the upper or lower jaw.

Extraoral X-rays:
Purpose: Providing an overall view of the oral and facial structures.
Techniques: Panoramic for a full-mouth view, cephalometric for orthodontic assessments, cone-beam computed tomography (CBCT) for detailed 3D imaging.

Bisecting Angle Technique:
Purpose: Capturing intraoral X-rays with minimal distortion.

Technique: Aligning the X-ray beam perpendicular to the bisector line between the long axis of the tooth and the film/sensor.

Parallel Technique:
Purpose: Minimizing image distortion and enhancing diagnostic accuracy.
Technique: Aligning the X-ray beam parallel to the long axis of the tooth and the film/sensor.

Safety Protocols:
Radiation Safety:
Lead Aprons and Thyroid Collars: Providing patients with protective gear to minimize radiation exposure to sensitive areas.
Limited Exposure Time: Keeping X-ray exposure time to the minimum required for diagnostic purposes.

Operator Safety:

Protective Barriers: Using lead-lined walls and doors in X-ray rooms to shield operators from radiation.

Personal Monitoring Devices: Regularly monitoring radiation exposure for dental staff through dosimeters.

Patient Education:
Informing Patients: Communicating the necessity and safety of dental X-rays for accurate diagnosis and treatment planning. Pregnancy Considerations: Implementing additional precautions for pregnant patients, such as shielding and discussing the benefits and risks.

Infection Control and Sterilization:

Instrument Sterilization:
Autoclave Use: Sterilizing dental instruments, including handpieces, scalers, and mirrors, to eliminate pathogens. Biological Monitoring: Regularly testing autoclave effectiveness through spore testing.

Surface Disinfection:
High-Touch Areas: Disinfecting surfaces, such as dental chairs, countertops, and light handles, between patients.

Barrier Techniques: Using disposable barriers on equipment and surfaces to prevent contamination.

Hand Hygiene:
Handwashing: Practicing thorough handwashing before and after patient contact.
Use of Hand Sanitizers: Using alcohol-based hand sanitizers when handwashing is not immediately possible.

Personal Protective Equipment (PPE):
Gloves, Masks, and Eyewear: Wearing appropriate PPE to protect against contact with blood, saliva, and other potentially infectious materials.
Proper Donning and Doffing: Ensuring correct procedures for putting on (donning) and taking off (doffing) PPE.

Patient Safety and Education:
Instrument Handling: Ensuring that instruments used during procedures are properly sterilized.
Patient Reassurance: Communicating infection control measures to patients to enhance confidence in the safety of dental care.
By adhering to strict X-ray techniques, safety protocols, and infection control measures, dental assistants contribute to maintaining a safe and sterile environment, safeguarding both patients and dental healthcare professionals.

6. Environmental Infection Control:
Aseptic Techniques: Implementing aseptic techniques to prevent contamination in the dental operatory.
Regular Disinfection: Routine disinfection of environmental surfaces, dental chairs, and equipment.

7. Sterile Instrument Handling:
Proper Packaging: Packaging sterilized instruments in a way that maintains sterility until use.
Segregation of Sterile and Non-Sterile Items: Ensuring clear separation between sterile and non-sterile items to prevent cross-contamination.

8. Waste Disposal:
Biomedical Waste Management: Proper disposal of biomedical waste, including used needles, contaminated materials, and disposable items.
Compliance with Regulations: Adhering to local regulations for biomedical waste disposal to protect public health and the environment.

9. Training and Education:
Continuous Training: Regular training for dental staff on infection control protocols and updates.

Patient Education: Educating patients on infection control measures to instill confidence in the safety of dental procedures.

10. Record Keeping:
Sterilization Logs: Maintaining detailed records of instrument sterilization cycles. Infection Control Protocols Documentation: Documenting adherence to infection control protocols for regulatory compliance.

11. Response to Infectious Incidents:
Emergency Protocols: Having clear protocols in place to respond to infectious incidents or exposures.
Contact Tracing: Conducting contact tracing and notifications when necessary to mitigate potential outbreaks.
In summary, infection control and sterilization are integral components of dental practice, ensuring the safety of both patients and dental healthcare providers. By meticulously following established

protocols, dental assistants play a pivotal role in maintaining a sterile and secure environment, fostering trust among patients and contributing to overall healthcare excellence.

Chapter five

Cross-contamination Prevention:

Hand Hygiene:
Thorough Handwashing: Ensuring all dental
personnel engage in thorough handwashing
before and after patient contact.
Use of Hand Sanitizers: Employing
alcohol-based hand sanitizers when
handwashing facilities are not immediately
accessible.

Personal Protective Equipment (PPE):
Gloves, Masks, and Eyewear: Utilizing
appropriate PPE to create a barrier between
the dental professional and potentially
infectious materials.
Regular Replacement of PPE: Changing
gloves and masks between patients to
prevent cross-contamination.

Instrument Handling:

Designated Sterile Zones: Establishing clearly defined sterile and non-sterile zones in the dental operatory.
Proper Instrument Passing: Ensuring instruments are passed in a way that minimizes the risk of contamination.
Surface Disinfection:

High-Touch Areas: Disinfecting surfaces, such as dental chairs, light handles, and countertops, between patients.
Barrier Techniques: Using disposable barriers on equipment and surfaces to prevent contamination.

Waste Management:
Proper Disposal: Ensuring proper disposal of contaminated materials in designated biomedical waste containers.
Segregation of Waste: Separating different categories of waste to avoid contamination.
Sterilization Procedures:

Autoclave Use:

Proper Loading: Loading instruments in a way that allows for effective steam penetration and sterilization.
Biological Monitoring: Regularly testing autoclave effectiveness through spore testing.

Instrument Packaging:
Correct Wrapping: Using appropriate sterilization wraps or pouches for different types of instruments.
Sealing and Labeling: Ensuring proper sealing and labeling to maintain sterility until use.

Sterilization Logs:
Documentation: Keeping detailed records of sterilization cycles, including date, time, and the contents of each cycle.
Monitoring Expiry Dates: Regularly checking and replacing sterilization indicators to ensure efficacy.

Ultrasonic Cleaning:
Instrument Preparation: Cleaning
instruments thoroughly before sterilization
to remove debris.
Safe Handling: Using ultrasonic cleaners in
accordance with manufacturer guidelines.

Dental Procedures and Techniques:
Infection Control During Procedures:
Aseptic Techniques: Implementing aseptic
techniques to minimize the risk of
introducing pathogens during dental
procedures.
Proper Instrument Handling: Ensuring
sterile instruments are used in accordance
with infection control protocols.

Patient Preparation:
Pre-procedural Rinses: Recommending or
providing antimicrobial mouth rinses to
reduce oral microbial load.
Isolation Techniques: Using dental dams or
other isolation methods to minimize
contamination during procedures.

Restorative Dentistry Procedures:
Cavity Preparation: Implementing techniques to minimize the generation of aerosols during cavity preparation.
Proper Handling of Restorative Materials: Ensuring the correct mixing and application of restorative materials to maintain their integrity.

Endodontic Procedures:
Aseptic Access Opening: Implementing aseptic techniques during access cavity preparation.
Instrument Handling in Root Canals: Using a sterile file for each canal and employing proper irrigation techniques.
Periodontal and Surgical Procedures:

Proper Tissue Management: Implementing techniques to control bleeding and maintain a clear surgical field.
Sterile Surgical Instruments: Ensuring all instruments used in surgical procedures are sterile and properly handled.

In conclusion, cross-contamination prevention, meticulous sterilization procedures, and adherence to infection control protocols are fundamental aspects of dental practice. These measures safeguard the well-being of both patients and dental healthcare providers, contributing to a safe and effective dental environment.

Chapter six

Chairside Assisting for Exams:

Patient Reception and Preparation:
Warm Welcome: Greeting patients warmly
and creating a comfortable atmosphere.
Update on Medical History: Reviewing and
updating the patient's medical history to
ensure accurate information.

Equipment and Room Setup:

Readiness of Instruments: Ensuring all
necessary instruments and materials are
prepared for the examination.
Comfortable Seating: Arranging the dental
chair for patient comfort and accessibility.

Assisting During Examination:
Instrument Transfer: Providing seamless
instrument transfer to the dentist during the
examination.

Suction Assistance: Assisting with suction to maintain a clear field of view for the dentist.

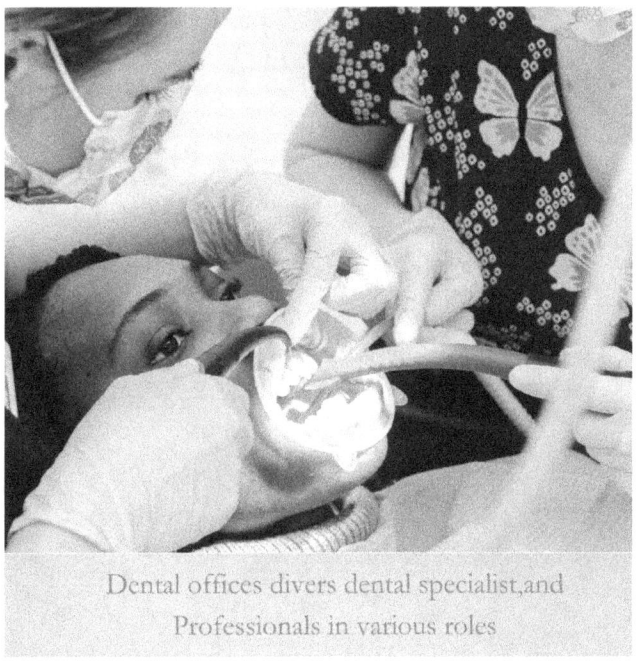

Dental offices divers dental specialist, and Professionals in various roles

Digital Imaging Assistance:
Positioning Sensors or Film: Ensuring proper placement of digital sensors or film for diagnostic imaging.
Patient Cooperation: Guiding patients on maintaining the correct position for imaging procedures.

Note-Taking and Documentation:
Recording Observations: Documenting the dentist's findings and observations during the examination.

Communication with the Dentist:

Communicating relevant information to the dentist for comprehensive patient care.

Restorative Dentistry Procedures:

Preparation for Restorative Procedures:

Patient Education: Explaining the planned restorative procedure to the patient, addressing any concerns.
Instrument Setup: Ensuring all necessary instruments and materials are prepared and organized.

Assisting During Tooth Preparation:

Retraction and Isolation: Assisting with the use of dental dams or retractors for proper isolation during tooth preparation.
Suction Assistance: Providing suction to maintain a dry field for the dentist.

Restorative Material Handling:
Mixing and Placement: Assisting with the proper mixing and placement of restorative materials.
Curing Assistance: Aiding in the use of curing lights for the setting of dental materials.

Post-Procedure Care:
Patient Instructions: Providing post-procedure care instructions to the patient.
Documentation: Recording details of the restorative procedure for patient records.

Dental Specialties:
Orthodontics:

Chairside Assistance in Orthodontic Exams: Aiding in the preparation and organization of instruments during orthodontic examinations.
Impressions and Mold Taking: Assisting with impressions for orthodontic appliances.

Oral Surgery:
Patient Preparation for Surgery: Assisting in pre-operative preparations, including positioning and comfort measures.
Instrument Transfer During Surgery: Ensuring the dentist has seamless access to required instruments during oral surgery procedures.

Pediatric Dentistry:

Child-Friendly Environment: Creating a welcoming and friendly atmosphere for pediatric patients.
Assisting During Pediatric Exams: Providing support during exams and procedures to alleviate anxiety.

Periodontics:
Assisting in Periodontal Exams: Aiding in the examination and documentation of periodontal conditions.
Maintenance of Sterile Field: Ensuring a sterile field during periodontal procedures.
In the realm of dental specialties, chairside assistants play a crucial role in supporting various dental procedures, contributing to the overall success of restorative and specialized treatments while prioritizing patient comfort and care.

Chapter seven

Orthodontics:

Orthodontic Examinations:
Patient Evaluation: Assessing the patient's oral health, facial structure, and alignment of teeth.
Radiographic Analysis: Assisting in taking and preparing X-rays for a comprehensive diagnostic evaluation.

Treatment Planning:

Impressions and Models: Aiding in the creation of impressions and models to plan orthodontic interventions.
Assisting in Record-Taking: Supporting the orthodontist in capturing detailed records, including photographs and cephalometric X-rays.

Bracket Placement and Adjustments:

Assisting During Bonding: Ensuring a smooth process for bonding brackets onto teeth.

Adjustment Appointments: Assisting with adjustments, wire changes, and other modifications during orthodontic visits.

Oral Hygiene Guidaa pp bynce: Providing instructions on maintaining oral hygiene with orthodontic appliances.

Comfort Measures: Offering guidance on managing discomfort associated with orthodontic treatment.

Oral Surgery:
Preoperative Preparation:
Patient Comfort: Assisting in ensuring patient comfort before oral surgery procedures.

Instrument Setup: Preparing and organizing instruments required for the specific surgical intervention.

Surgical Assistance:
Suction and Retraction: Aiding with suction to maintain a clear surgical field and providing retraction support.
Instrument Transfer: Ensuring efficient and sterile transfer of instruments during surgery.

Postoperative Care:
Patient Monitoring: Observing and monitoring patients in the postoperative period.
Post-Surgical Instructions: Assisting in conveying postoperative care instructions to patients and caregivers.

Documentation:
Record-Keeping: Documenting details of the surgical procedure for patient records and future reference.
Communication with the Surgical Team: Facilitating effective communication within the surgical team.

Pediatric Dentistry:
Child-Friendly Environment:
Welcoming Atmosphere: Creating a warm and friendly environment to alleviate pediatric anxiety.
Use of Child-Centric Language: Communicating in a manner suitable for children to enhance understanding.

Patient Cooperation:
Behavior Management Techniques: Assisting in the application of behavior management strategies during exams and treatments.
Positive Reinforcement: Encouraging and positively reinforcing cooperative behavior.

Preventive Care:
Fluoride Applications: Assisting in the application of fluoride treatments for cavity prevention.
Sealant Placement: Aiding in the placement of dental sealants to protect vulnerable areas of teeth.

Education for Parents:
Parental Guidance: Providing parents with guidance on oral hygiene practices and preventive care.
Nutritional Counseling: Offering advice on a child's diet and its impact on oral health.

Dental Emergencies:
Patient Triage:
Assessment of Urgency: Determining the urgency of the dental emergency.
Immediate Comfort Measures: Providing immediate relief for pain and discomfort.

Emergency Protocols:
Communication with Emergency Services: Coordinating with emergency services when required.
First Aid Procedures: Administering basic first aid for dental emergencies.

Documentation:
Recording Incident Details: Documenting the nature of the dental emergency, actions taken, and patient response.
Communication with Dentist: Conveying pertinent information to the dentist for further evaluation.

Follow-Up Care:

Post-Emergency Instructions: Providing clear instructions for follow-up care and further treatment.

Scheduling Appointments: Assisting in scheduling necessary follow-up appointments for continued care.

In each of these dental specialties and emergency situations, chairside assistants play a vital role in ensuring a smooth and supportive dental experience for patients while facilitating the work of the dental team.

Chapter eight

Common Emergencies:

Toothache:
Cause: Dental decay, infection, or trauma.
Symptoms: Severe pain, swelling.
Immediate Response: Provide pain relief, rinse with warm water, and schedule a dental appointment.

Knocked-Out Tooth:
Cause: Trauma or injury.
Immediate Response: Retrieve the tooth, hold it by the crown (not the root), rinse gently, and attempt to re-implant. If not possible, store in milk and seek immediate dental care.

Broken or Fractured Tooth:
Cause: Trauma or biting on hard objects.
Immediate Response: Rinse mouth with warm water, apply a cold compress to reduce swelling, and see a dentist promptly.

Object Caught Between Teeth:
Cause: Food or foreign object lodged between teeth.
Immediate Response: Gently try to dislodge with dental floss, avoiding sharp objects. If unsuccessful, seek dental assistance.

Response and First Aid:

Toothache:
Response: Assess the severity of pain and swelling.
First Aid: Provide over-the-counter pain relief, recommend warm saltwater rinses, and schedule a dental appointment.

Knocked-Out Tooth:
Response: Remain calm and retrieve the tooth.
First Aid: Attempt to re-implant the tooth if possible, store in milk or saline if not, and seek immediate dental care.

Broken or Fractured Tooth:
Response: Address pain and swelling.
First Aid: Rinse the mouth, apply a cold compress, and visit a dentist for evaluation and possible restoration.

Object Caught Between Teeth:
Response: Assess discomfort and attempt self-removal.
First Aid: Gently use dental floss to remove the object, avoiding damage to the gums or teeth. Seek professional assistance if unsuccessful.

Dental Assisting Certification:
Education and Training:
Formal Education: Completion of a recognized dental assisting program.
Clinical Training: Hands-on training in dental procedures, radiography, and chairside assisting.

Certification Examination:

National Certification: Successful completion of a nationally recognized certification exam.

Verification of Competency: Demonstration of proficiency in key dental assisting skills.

Continuing Education:

Requirement for Renewal: Regular completion of continuing education credits for certification renewal.
Stay Current: Keeping abreast of industry advancements and changes through ongoing education.
Code of Ethics and Professionalism:

Adherence to Standards: Following a code of ethics and professional conduct.
Patient Confidentiality: Maintaining strict confidentiality regarding patient information.

Career Advancement:
Opportunities for Growth: Certification opens doors to various dental specialties and career advancement.
Recognition of Competency: Certification serves as a testament to a dental assistant's competence and dedication to professional standards.

In summary, a dental assisting certification signifies the completion of rigorous education and training, adherence to professional standards, and ongoing commitment to excellence in patient care. Dental assistants with certifications are valuable contributors to the dental healthcare team.

Educational institutions, classrooms, and workshops

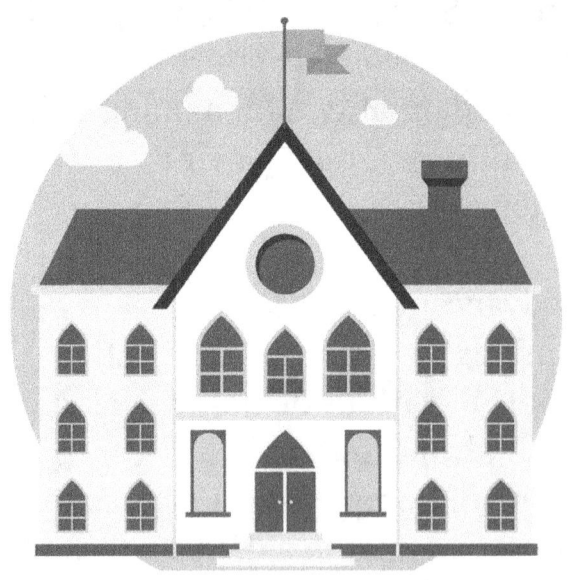

Chapter nine

Educational Requirements:

High School Diploma or Equivalent:
Prerequisite: Attainment of a high school
diploma or equivalent.
Foundation: Provides the foundational
knowledge required for pursuing further
education in dental assisting.

Formal Dental Assisting Program:
Accredited Program: Enrollment in an
accredited dental assisting program.
Curriculum: Comprehensive coursework
covering dental anatomy, radiography,
chairside procedures, and infection control.

Clinical Training:

Hands-On Experience: Practical, clinical
training in a dental setting.

Supervised Practice: Application of theoretical knowledge in real-world scenarios under the guidance of experienced dental professionals.

Certification Exams:

Eligibility Criteria:
Completion of Education: Fulfillment of educational requirements from an accredited dental assisting program.
Clinical Experience: Minimum hours of supervised clinical experience.
National Board Dental Assisting

Examination (NBDHE):
Content: Comprehensive exam covering various aspects of dental assisting.
Passing Score: Attainment of a passing score to demonstrate competency.

State-Specific Exams:
Varied Requirements: Some states may have additional or specific exams for certification.

Licensure: Successful completion of state-specific exams may contribute to obtaining a dental assisting license.

Renewal and Continuing Education:
Maintenance of Certification: Regular renewal of certification through continuing education.
Stay Current: Engaging in ongoing professional development to stay current with industry advancements.

Chapter ten

Professional Development:

Continuing Education:
Requirement for Renewal: Mandatory completion of continuing education credits for certification renewal.
Varied Topics: Courses covering new technologies, infection control updates, and emerging trends in dental assisting.

Specialized Training and Certifications:
Expanded Functions: Pursuit of additional certifications for expanded functions like coronal polishing or pit and fissure sealants.
Orthodontic or Surgical Assisting: Specialized training for those interested in orthodontics or oral surgery.

Professional Memberships:

Joining Associations: Becoming a member of dental assisting associations.
Networking: Opportunities for networking, mentorship, and access to resources for professional growth.

Advanced Degrees or Specializations:

Pursuing Higher Education: Seeking advanced degrees for career advancement.
Dental Specializations: Pursuing specialization in areas like dental hygiene or dental laboratory technology.

Career Advancement Opportunities: Supervisory Roles: Advancement to supervisory or managerial positions within a dental practice.

Teaching and Training: Opportunities for teaching or training future dental assistants.

In conclusion, the journey of a dental assistant involves meeting educational requirements, successfully passing certification exams, and engaging in continuous professional development. This commitment ensures a high standard of care and opens doors to various career advancement opportunities within the dental field.

Conclusion

Continuing Education:

Regulatory Requirements:
Mandatory Credits: Fulfilling continuing education requirements to maintain certification.
Stay Informed: Staying abreast of changes in regulations, guidelines, and best practices.

Specialized Training:

Advanced Certifications: Pursuing specialized certifications in areas like radiography, infection control, or dental materials.
Advanced Procedures: Gaining expertise in new dental technologies and procedures through targeted education.

Workshops and Seminars:

Interactive Learning: Participating in workshops and seminars for hands-on training.
Networking Opportunities: Connecting with professionals and staying engaged in the dental community.

Career Opportunities:
Expanded Roles:
Orthodontic Assistant: Assisting in orthodontic procedures and working closely with orthodontists.
Oral Surgery Assistant: Supporting oral surgeons in various surgical procedures.

Teaching and Training:
Educational Roles: Transitioning into roles as dental assisting educators.
Training Programs: Instructing new dental assistants or leading training programs.

Administrative Positions:
Office Manager: Advancing into managerial roles within dental practices.

Administrative Support: Contributing to the efficient running of dental offices.

Research and Product Development:
Industry Opportunities: Exploring roles in
dental product development or research.
Consulting: Providing expertise to dental
product companies.

Mobile Dentistry:
Community Outreach: Participating in
mobile dental clinics for community
outreach.
Access to Care: Increasing access to dental
services for underserved populations.
Conclusion and Future Trends in Dental

Assisting:
Technological Integration:
Digital Dentistry: Embracing digital tools
for charting, imaging, and treatment
planning.

Telehealth: Integrating telehealth solutions
for patient consultations and follow-ups.

Infection Control and Safety:
Heightened Measures: Continued emphasis on infection control, especially in response to global health concerns.
Advanced Sterilization Technologies: Adoption of advanced sterilization methods for instruments.

Expanded Scope of Practice:
Legislative Changes: Advocating for expanded functions and responsibilities for dental assistants.
Collaborative Care Models: Collaborating closely with other healthcare professionals for comprehensive patient care.

Patient-Centered Care:
Communication Skills: Enhancing communication skills for effective patient education.
Cultural Competence: Developing cultural competence for diverse patient populations.

Sustainability in Dentistry:
Eco-Friendly Practices: Integration of environmentally sustainable practices in dental offices.
Reducing Waste: Implementing strategies to minimize waste generation in dental procedures.
In conclusion, the future of dental assisting holds exciting opportunities for career growth, advanced education, and embracing emerging trends in technology and patient care. As the field evolves, dental assistants will continue to play a vital role in providing high-quality oral healthcare.

Opportunities:
Enroll in relevant workshops, seminars, or online courses to stay current with the latest advancements in dental assisting.

Diversify Your Skill Set:
Pursue specialized certifications or training programs to expand your expertise and open doors to new career opportunities.

Join dental assisting associations, attend conferences, and connect with peers to build a strong professional network and stay informed about industry trends.

Consider Career Advancement Paths:
Evaluate potential career paths within dental assisting, such as orthodontic or oral surgery assisting, administrative roles, or teaching positions.

Embrace Technology in Dentistry:
Stay informed about emerging technologies in dentistry, such as digital tools and telehealth solutions, and explore how they can enhance your practice.

Advocate for Legislative Changes:
Get involved in advocating for expanded functions for dental assistants to contribute to the evolution of the profession.

Prioritize Patient-Centered Care:
Enhance your communication skills and
cultural competence to provide
patient-centered care and foster positive
relationships with diverse patient
populations.
Contribute to Sustainable Dentistry:
Explore eco-friendly practices and waste
reduction strategies within your dental
practice to contribute to sustainability
efforts in dentistry.

Set Professional Development Goals:
Develop a plan for ongoing professional
development, including obtaining advanced
certifications and pursuing higher education
if applicable.

Stay Informed About Industry Trends:
Regularly read industry publications, attend
webinars, and engage with reputable
sources to stay informed about the latest
trends and future directions in dental
assisting.

Remember, taking proactive steps toward professional growth and staying engaged with industry developments will not only enhance your career but also contribute to the overall advancement of dental assisting as a vital component of oral healthcare.

www.ingramcontent.com/pod-product-compliance
Lightning Source LLC
Chambersburg PA
CBHW062356290526
45794CB00005B/2257